Ayurvedic Wellness: Basic Ayurveda For Westerners

WELLNESS COACHING SERIES:

LIFESTYLE TRANSFORMATION WITH AYURVEDA

By James Adler

Copyright James Adler© 2014

www.facebook.com/HolisticWellnessBooks

All rights reserved. No part of this publication may be reproduced, stored in a retrieval system, or transmitted, in any form or by any means, electronic, mechanical, photocopying, recording or otherwise, without the prior written permission of the author and the publishers.

The scanning, uploading, and distribution of this book via the Internet or via any other means without the permission of the author is illegal and punishable by law. Please purchase only authorized electronic editions, and do not participate in or encourage electronic piracy of copyrighted materials.

Table of Contents

<u>Introduction:</u> Ayurvedic Lifestyle and Wellness

Discover what Ayurveda can do for you and transform your life…5

<u>Chapter 1:</u> My Journey to Understanding Holistic Balance

How I managed to stop the vicious circle of addictions thanks to Ayurveda. My studies in Kerala…8

<u>Chapter 2:</u> The Great Elements and Ayurvedic Wellness

Understand how Ayurveda works. The Ayurvedic Philosophy is not difficult at all! Immerse yourself in this holistic approach step by step…13

<u>Chapter 3:</u> The Three Doshas: Different Strokes for Different Folks

Everyone is different and Ayurveda has some answers for you. Learn more about yourself and correct those imbalances. Create your lifestyle according to your dosha…19

<u>Chapter 4:</u> True Healthcare and Real Treatment

Discover Ayurvedic Natural Remedies and Therapies for Balance and Wellness!…30

<u>Chapter 5:</u> Ayurvedic Recipes for Wellness and Balance…40

I love cooking. In this chapter I have gathered the best of Ayurvedic recipes I learned in Kerala. After learning your prevalent dosha you will be able to discover wellness and health via balanced, Ayurvedic body and mind nutrition. Enjoy!...40

<u>Conclusion:</u> Ayurveda is a Science of Life. Are you willing to apply it?...61

Introduction: Ayurvedic Lifestyle and Wellness

I want to thank you for purchasing the book: "Ayurveda for Beginners: Ayurvedic Lifestyle for Westerners".

I have written this book in order to share the wonderful healthcare system known as Ayurveda. It is not a healthcare plan that treats your physical and emotional symptoms. It is a method that <u>rebalances</u> the body and mind with the world around you.

With Ayurveda you will learn what to eat, what not to eat, and what to stay away from environmentally and emotionally. You will eventually receive an individualized plan to attack illness and put all things back into balance, according to your specific needs.

You can say goodbye to stress, addiction, illness and mental cloudiness, all by rebalancing your lifestyle just as I did. No longer will you look at curing the symptom, you will be trying to find the source: the part of you that is out of balance.

It sounds easy, and it is. I wrote this book as to give beginners an overall idea on what Ayurveda is all about. It is intended as a guide to get you started. As westerners, we do not always have a grasp on such things. We get sucked into day to day life, and sometimes lose sight of the big picture. It is my hope that you will see the use of Ayurvedic medicine to restore balance to your life.

Say "no" from now on to standard toxic drugs and medicines that only perpetuate imbalance and treat symptoms. Instead, I hope you embrace a new, ancient approach to healthcare, and restore your body/mind balance in order to find true health and wellness.

Disclaimer:

A physician has not written the information in this book. Although the Ayurvedic therapies are generally safe to use, if you suffer from any serious medical condition, are pregnant, or on medication you should consult your doctor (preferably a doctor who specializes in oriental medicine) first to see if you can apply it. It is also advisable that you visit a qualified Ayurvedic Doctor so that you can obtain a highly personalized treatment for your case, especially if you want to make Ayurveda a part of your lifestyle. This book is for informational and educational purposes only.

All information in this book has been carefully researched and checked for factual accuracy. However, the author and publishers make no warranty, expressed or implied, that the information contained herein is appropriate for every individual, situation or purpose, and assume no responsibility for errors or omission. The reader assumes the risk and full responsibility for all actions, and the author will not be held liable for any loss or damage, whether consequential, incidental, and special or otherwise that may result from the information presented in this publication.

Chapter 1 My Journey to Understanding Balance

Most Westerners have heard of Ayurveda, yet are not exactly sure what it is. It sounds mystical and magical; and it is. Yet, it is also a very real and holistic way of approaching health and wellness by developing a solid mind and body balance.

My name is James. I, probably like yourself, had heard of Ayurveda but had no real understanding of the practicality and usefulness of it. I thought it was a magical religion. As I found out, it was actually magical in fixing my life, and the most amazing healthcare plan I have ever signed up for.

In my younger years, I partied non-stop. I was also a serious workaholic. I ate what I needed to, in a pinch. My life was a constant circle of addiction (drugs, alcohol and work). I was stressed to the maximum. I had to have a drink or a smoke in order to not let the stress of my job get to me. Yet, those drinks and drugs would all catch up with me on Monday morning.

I hated my life. I despised my job; working 9-9 as a manager for a marketing company. I even despised my employees (yeah, not a great manager). I was always on edge and used the alcohol and drugs to balance myself out, or so I thought.

One day, a friend suggested I take up yoga. I thought yoga was for girls. Eventually, weeks later I gave in. I signed up for a class and went. That was really the beginning of the rest of my life. I remember it clearly, I was 27 and it was a spring morning. My yoga instructor was a male, John. He seemed to like me and spent some extra time answering the questions I had; I wanted to know about this balancing act he called Ayurveda.

Slowly I began studying and really learning about it in my spare time. Everything finally made sense. The things I had been doing to keep the balance in my life, were actually causing imbalances. I had taken the wrong approach.

I saved up money for several months. My enlightenment led me to go to India. I had to immerse myself in Eastern Ayurveda. I had to live and breathe it. I spent a year there; traveling and taking courses and workshops in Kerala. I knew I needed more massive change in my life. I wanted the ultimate balance in order to achieve optimum health and wellness.

I decided that a marketing career was definitely not for me. I wanted to help others rebalance their lives and bodies just as I had. Ayurveda is not too good to be true, and I wanted to help other individuals see that and experience it as well.

I am now a life coach. I am not an Ayurvedic practitioner, but I always add an Ayurvedic touch to all of my guidance. After all, I cannot help it, I truly have been transformed. It comes across in every aspect of my life as it should. Join me as I help to enlighten you with the contents of this book.

Ayurveda originates from an oral tradition that was eventually put into ancient Indian manuscripts known as the Vedas. They are at least 5000 years old. Ayurveda could quite possibly be the oldest life-science based upon what could be the oldest human writings. The name "Ayurveda" comes from the Sanskrit language and is broken down as "ayus," meaning life, and "ved," meaning knowledge. It is the science of life and living and all that it encompasses; which makes it applicable to any era.

Our lives are a combination of our souls (Atma), our minds (Mana), our five senses that we use to process the world (Indriyan), and our bodies (Sharira).

Health is a lifelong continuous process that we all participate in. It is affected by, and has an effect on our physical, emotional, mental, social and universal state.

Everything in Ayurveda is intertwined. It is a holistic, cohesive system of true health care. In practicing this science, your objective is to balance emotional state, mental state and the physical state in order to achieve maximum health. You cannot be physically well without being emotionally well. You cannot achieve optimal mental health without being emotionally or physically healthy (and vice-versa).

Ayurveda followers have to include all aspects of life in order to be truly healthy through a delicate balance. These areas include, but are not limited to: eating, standard of living, exercising, detoxifying, sleeping, and the brain. Ayurveda blends and enhances everyday activities and lifestyle habits in order to enrich health and prevent illnesses of the spirit, mind and body. The areas of enhancement include (also not limited to): what is eaten, meditating, practicing yoga, exercising, using herbs, massage, color, aroma therapy, and musical therapies, and having a different perspective about life in general.

Ayurveda provides us with personal, individualized suggestions. It covers everything in our lifestyles: from our activities, to specific therapies to battle disease. It truly is an ancient all-inclusive personalized healthcare program, so different in so many ways from the western version of health care that uses a "one-prescription-fits-most" approach.

Chapter 2 The Great Elements

Ayurveda not only focuses on the mind and body but the world around us. The five elements of the universe are part of the balancing act that is the key to the Ayurveda healthcare system. We use these elements to pin point the feeble and resilient aspects of ourselves and then utilize its harmonizing elements in our eating, routines and surroundings.

In Ayurveda these five elements are the foundation of life. Universally, all things are made up of these five elements. When you are able to comprehend principal elements relating to yourself and your environment, you can somewhat figure out how they will influence you and be able to find means to use contrasting elements to achieve a better balance.

They are called the *Pancha Maha Bhuta* in Sanskrit, meaning the five great elements. They are listed in a specific order from the more elusive and imperceptible to the more substantial, tangible and unrefined. They are Ether (Akasha), Air (Vayu), Fire (Agni), Water (Jala), and Earth (Prithvi). We, as Westerners need to understand that each element is not literal, they are representative of things and energies that collaborate in the universe. We have been trained to see water as just that, water. But when broken down Ayurvedically, water has particles in it that are earth. There are molecules present that are made up of atoms; the area between the atoms is ether. The temperature of warmer water is related to fire. As evaporation occurs, air is also interconnected. Sure, running water is water, but in Ayurveda it is much more than that.

1. **Ether/Askasha**

   Askasha is the most seemingly abstract and the most delicate element. It has a certain magical aspect about it. It is all-encompassing, ever-present and powerful. It is the place where everything exists and all that is in between. It is one thing that we cannot experience through our five senses. It is virtually limitless. It was the primary manifestation of awareness in nature, so its importance is held in high regard in the Ayurvedic community. In our bodies it is characterized by the area between molecules and our spirit. Ether oversees the perception of sound and everything to do with the mouth and sound from the vocal cords. This makes sense as sound moves through ether.

   Attributes: transparent, weightless, flowing, and infinite.

2. Air/Vayu

Vayu's main cause is motion. Whenever there is movement we know that air is there. Vayu means wind or air, but in Ayurveda it means much more. It cannot be defined by a single word. Moving through the continuum of elements away from ether and more toward the tangible, air is where we take on an objective; an indication of where we want to go in the direction of. It is sometimes unpredictable and can easily take an alternate path. In our bodies it displays as the energy in the body (the nervous system, tissue and cell function, and the development of gas). Air oversees every sense; most importantly that of touch and the use of the hands to provide, accept, and move objects.

Attributes: traveling, waterless, wispy, chilly, coarse, and elusive

3. Fire/Agni

Agni is all about change and breakdown/absorption. All molecules exchange heat when transforming. In our bodies it is demonstrated as astuteness and understanding, regulation of body temperatures, digestion and metabolism, and the liver's processes. The blood carries fire in the body. If the blood does not travel to an area, that area will become cold.

This is where we concentrate energy into a concept or objective and utilize our fire to begin bringing it into fruition. Fire oversees vision and motion of the legs (as we move toward our goals).

Attributes: warm/hot, sudden, waterless, indirect, light

4. Water/Jala

Jala's main concentration is on transference and is a solvent. In our bodies it is represented by plasma and lymph, transporting nourishment through our bodies and toxins out of our bodies. Jala is the river of life. Moving even closer toward the tangible, water is where an idea we are fixated on requires nutrition in order to come to fruition. Water is the element responsible for taste and breeding by way of the sex organs.

Attributes: blunt, cool, liquescent, smooth, slippery, and greasy

5. Earth/Prithvi

Structure is the main purpose of Prithvi. Solidity, longevity and firmness all signify that supremacy of earth is at play. It is the cornerstone of the planet. It provides all living beings with structure, nutrition and accommodations. It is seen in the body as the dense formations that we are made up of: skeleton, muscle, tendon, nail, hair, teeth and membranes. Prithvi is the point where awareness becomes a tangible substance. It rules our ability to smell and excretion of waste from the body.

Attributes: dense, blunt, continuous, weighty, and durable.

These five elements nourish and support life when they are kept balanced. Alternatively, unbalanced elements will cause illness, discomfort and chaos. When we are able to comprehend the way the elements work and how they present themselves in the body, it is easy to pinpoint and prescribe the proper treatment for an excess of a certain element. Such as, anxiety's effect on the body's nervous system. Anxiety intensifies Vayu (air) in the physiological system. The excess of air would cause and imbalance that could manifest itself as dry-skin or feeling cold. Utilizing the Ayurvedic elemental arrangement, we would find an opposite element (like water) to bring harmony back into the body. We can prescribe ourselves things that are associated with water (Jala): affection, melodiousness, exercise to music, or good the use of healthy fats (internally and externally).

These are just examples of things that we can do to minimize and over-ride the amount of air in order to get back to a balanced state free of worry and anxiety. This is only a small example, but as you can see, it is easily done with Ayurvedic treatments that are both tangible and physical in combination with more spiritual and elusive methods.

Chapter 3 The Three Doshas: Different Strokes for Different Folks

If you are like me you have probably wondered what makes people different. Why are some people hyper and social, while others are introverted and graceful? Why do some people seem to be able to eat all day long without a problem when others can barely choke down a meal? Why are some people always care-free, when many people are constantly stressed? Yes, some of these traits are genetic, but what about the things that are unique to each individual? Ayurveda gives insight to these differences thanks to three energies called Doshas. They are found in every person's body and brain.

The three Doshas are responsible for all bodily functions and thought processes and how they are related to the world around us. When broken down, they will give each individual a process of treatment and prevention that will ultimately lead to holistic health in order to get the most out of life.

The three Doshas

Vata: traits of ether and air.

Pitta: traits of fire and water

Kapha: traits water and earth

When practicing Ayurveda, the goal is to keep all of these in balance in order to maintain homeostasis. They are regulatory so when they fall out of balance disease and illness can ravage the mind and body.

Every human being comes into this world with a different combination of doshas; the ratio of each is unique to each individual. We have them from the second we are formed in the womb and will carry them throughout our lives. Most people have one or a combination of two doshas that dominate their being. We will have those physiological and psychological tendencies embedded in us, thanks to our dominant doshas.

Our doshas will be in one of 3 conditions:

1. Balance: doshas are the way that they are naturally supposed to be.
2. Increase: there is a surplus of a dosha.
3. Decrease: there is a dosha lacking in quantity.

Having an increase of a dosha will cause the most amounts of problems because imbalance will be more widespread. This can be caused by not eating properly and by lifestyle or emotional stressors. It is easy to regain your equilibrium once you have an idea of your dominant doshas and their tendencies. You will be able to compliment your internal and external environments.

Most problems of decreased or increased doshas are associated with the dominant dosha. Perhaps you are a Pitta who has chronic indigestion. Eating more alkalizing foods will help you to prevent the problem and also help your Pitta dosha to thrive and be in balance. A key to Ayurveda is that if you add the same thing to your problem, you will make it worse. You diffuse and prevent problems by adding the opposite in order to be balanced.

Here is a little more information on each dosha:

Vata

Elements: Air/Ether

- Vata's energy is that of moving (movement). It is the driving force behind all bodily processes. It oversees our life-force and provides mobility to Kapha and Pitta.
- Someone who is Vata usually has a slight build. Their thinking is quick and they may change their minds often. They appear to be impulsive

and volatile. When stressed, Vatas experience anxiety and become agitated.

- Vatas are usually very active and artistic. They are great communicators and can express their thinking and emotions clearly. Vatas are able to think very quickly.

- When there is an imbalance with Vata, there is no hiding it. They can and will experience anxiety and become agitated easily. They experience physical problems such as dryness of the skin and are easily constipated.

- Vata is based in the colon, upper legs, skeleton, joints, ears, membranes, mind and nerves. It oversees all things moving in the body such as: inhaling, exhaling, nerve impulses, circulatory system, digestion, greater body movement, female period, bowel movements and urination.

- Mentally, it takes care of creativeness, ability to change thought processes quickly, communicating, and the capacity to think fast.

You can help to keep Vata balanced by:
- Eating foods appropriate for Vata
- Consuming foods in a calm atmosphere
- Spend time in nature

- Have a routine everyday
- Get enough sleep while it is dark
- Meditate everyday
- Exercise regularly, enlisting activities such as yoga, walk, or swim

Vata can become imbalanced by:
- Ingesting foods that aggravate Vata
- Eating while being nervous or unhappy
- Having meals on the go
- Alcoholic beverages, coffee-drinks, tea (black)
- Tobacco smoke
- Not having a regular routine
- Falling asleep too late in the night

Pitta

- Elements: Water/Fire
- Pitta's energy is that of assimilation and absorption in the body. It operates through the liquids that make these processes possible. It is

closer in relation to Fire, but these fluids are behind the Water aspect of Pitta.

- Pittas normally have a medium build. Their thought processes are organized and they make decisions easily. They come across as forceful and passionate, extreme and intense. When pressured they may become suddenly very irritated.

- Pitta people, when in balance, have jubilant personalities and are daring and driven. Pitta are very intelligent and are able to think quickly.

- When out of balance, Pitta will quickly become angry. They will be centered on their own ego. This is their Fire showing itself to the extreme. It is easy for their good qualities to be completely overshadowed. Their arrogance will push people away and they will become jaded. This imbalance will manifest physically with different types of: infections, fevers, skin outbreaks, sores, indigestion, pre-mature balding or greying of the hair, and chronic-inflammation.

- Pitta is prevalent in the intestine and gut. It is also located in livers, spleens, and pancreases. It is also found in fluid like plasma and sweat. It is responsible for warmth in the body and is the source of energy in digestion. Pitta is in charge of all converting and transforming that takes place in the brain and the body. Emotionally, Pitta is responsible for happiness, bravery, strength of the will, rage, jealousy, and how emotions are triggered by the mind. Last but not least, Pitta is the radiance of the brain.

To keep Pitta balanced:

- Eat a diet rich in foods that balance Pitta
- Dine in peace
- Do not drink stimulants or ingest them at all (fuel to the fire)
- Take up calming hobbies; especially those involving nature
- Meditate on a regular basis
- Exercise by doing something peaceful like take a walk or swim

Pitta becomes unbalanced by:
- Working too much
- Drinking alcoholic beverages, coffee-drinks, and tea (black)
- Smoking tobacco or using drugs
- Engaging in too much competition
- Eating Pitta aggravating foods

Kapha

- Elements: Water/Earth

- People who are Kapha have the energy of lubricating and building. It provides the physical aspect of our bodies and the flowing operation of all of its components. It is the adhesive that holds everything together and lubricates the physique.

- Physically speaking, Kaphas are usually more heavy-set. When functioning at their finest, Kaphas are tranquil and easy-going. They come across as very stress-free. When Kaphas are stressed or pressured they shut down, becoming very quiet.

- Kapha takes up home in the upper torso, throat, cranium, lungs, lymph nodes, fat and connective tissues, and in the tendons/ligaments. Kapha is responsible for moisturizing the foods that they eat, giving substance to their tissue, lubricating their joints, and stockpiling energy. Kapha is associated with the cool bodily fluids. In the mind, Kapha oversees affection, tolerance and forgiveness, gluttony, and mental apathy. Kapha can help rebalance Vata and Pitta.

- Water can be a good thing, but too much of it and you will flood your body unnecessarily. This is what happens when there is a Kapha imbalance. The body becomes physically overwhelmed with fluid. It can affect the mind as well, making thoughts and emotions cloudy. Imbalanced Kaphas are prone to becoming obese and problems that stem from too much mucous. Sweet, peaceful Kapha can turn into a lazy, depressed, unmotivated individual.

To keep Kapha balanced:

- Eat a diet that is full of Kapha foods
- Eat where you feel loved
- Stay away from extravagance and relaxation in excess
- Remember to practice and focus on non-attachment
- Self-evaluate and redirect emotions on a regular basis
- Take up introspective activities: meditation and writing/journaling
- Do not allow others to walk all over you
- Get enough sleep as early in the evening as possible: no naps

Kapha becomes unbalanced by:

- Eating foods that are not designed for Kaphas
- Eating too much of anything
- Emotional eating (comfort foods, sweets, etc.)
- Not exercising
- Staying inside all of the time
- Not staying intellectually challenged

In my life the differences between the doshas made perfect sense. I had always been confused why my best friend and I would react so opposite under the same exact circumstances. I just thought that it was because she was a female, or because she had been raised differently. This was not the case at all, come to find out, after I learned all about the different doshas.

Jane, my best friend, would constantly stay in relationships that were damaging and unhealthy for years at a time. She knew that they were bad but would not find a reason to cut it off. She would stick around long after the relationship was dead. I, on the other hand, was quick to move on after a relationship with a woman would become stagnant, let alone damaging.

Jane also had the tendency to shut down when she would get stressed out and over-whelmed. Instead of attacking her problems, she would literally hide from them, pretending they were not there. This would only compound problems. I could not figure out why in the world she would continually do this, seeing the same terrible result every time.

After I learned all about each dosha, I was able to understand that these were her psychological responses. She was a Kapha to a tee; even her body type. Once I was able to share with her information regarding her dosha, she was able to take steps necessary to re-balance her state when it became in excess. She was also able to battle, head on, the way she would react to things. As they say, "knowing is half the battle."

Each human being has a different combination of the doshas. Once you figure out your dosha type, you can figure out how to balance your mind and body using different diet and lifestyle adaptations.
Understanding and working with your dosha type will enable you to achieve optimum health and wellness.

Chapter 4 True Healthcare and Real Treatment

The Ayurvedic healthcare system is far different from Western medicinal healthcare systems. Western medicine is based upon treating a symptom with a chemical. It does not usually focus on finding the true source of the problem, it also does not take into consideration the differences of each person; both physical and emotional. Ayurveda uses quite a bit of individual analysis and takes into account the differences in each person. It utilizes therapies, instead of toxic drugs, to restore balance to the individual: both physically and psychologically. Ayurveda recognizes the individuality in humans and prescribes therapies that will keep the body and mind in balance; the only way to achieve holistic wellness.

Instead of drugs, a typical Ayurvedic prescription for a condition would consist of foods to restore balance and therapies to help the process along. Typical Ayurvedic prescribed therapies are: yoga, meditation, detoxes and cleansing the body, best exercise for that person, massage, ingestion of herbs, and many more. There are many people/practitioners available to help prescribe and preform therapies.

Some Ayurvedic therapies can be administered easily at home. Here are 5 of the ailments that Ayurvedic home remedies can help with and a few of the remedies available to try:

1. Asthma/tamak swas: inflammation of the airway that leads to coughing, wheezing, and lack of air flow to the lungs.

   Remedies

   - ½ tsp. of ginger (grate) is boiled in milk, then ¼ tsp. turmeric is stirred in. Drink 2x/day

   - Ginger tea and 3 smashed garlic cloves. Drink as needed.

   - Inhale steam and rub warm sesame oil and salt on chest to break up mucous

Avoid: Heavy foods, dairy, fried foods, pickled foods, beans/legumes. Do not eat to engorgement. Dust, cold air and smoke should not be inhaled.

2. Constipation: problems with elimination are most likely an imbalance of vata. Vata out of balance can cause dryness in the body and therefore problems with movement within the body.

   Remedies:

- Drink more water in the mornings, beginning with 2 or 3 and work your way up to 7. Keep the water in a copper vessel at night.

- Soak figs and drink the water they were sitting in (overnight). Eat when you wake up. Then soak more and eat at night. 4 Figs/2xday

- 2 tsp castor oil by mouth right before sleeping.

Avoid: Foods that are fried, refined sugar and bleached flour items, dairy, and anything processed. Limit dry foods, cold foods, and processed foods. Avoid eating too much.

3. Sinusitis/pinas: inflamed tissue of the sinuses. It causes sneezing, congestion, headaches, and makes it hard to breathe.

    Remedies:

- Bring down internal swelling by inhaling steam. Add cloves or mint to the water you are using. 15 min 2x/day while sick and then 1x/week as prevention

- 1 tsp. fresh ginger juice mixed with 1 tsp. honey 2x/day

- 5 peeled and crushed garlic cloves will alleviate congestion

Avoid: Sweets, cold or greasy food, chocolate, and cold beverages. Lack of sleep.

4. Eczema/asyicharchika: a skin condition where patches of skin become red, swell, itch and are dry and flaky. It flares up when the immune system has an imbalance.

   Remedies:

- Boil thirty margosa leaves in five cups water for twenty min, cool and then apply and wash area with the water.

- 1 tsp licorice (root powdered) mixed with a tad sesame oil, warm mix in a pan and then put on the problem areas. Use a bandage to cover for 4 hours 2x/day

Avoid: greasy or spicy foods. Stay away from humidity and warm weather. Do not wear man-made fibers in your clothes. No caffeinated beverages or preservatives.

5. Anorexia/aruchi: a complete lack of appetite, even when hunger is present and food is needed and available. It can be chosen, or come about because of an inactive lifestyle, too much stress, or bad eating habits.

Remedies:

- Mix ¼ tsp. juiced ginger, ¼ tsp. juiced lime with a pinch rock salt. Drink 2x/day before eating.

- Mix up equal amounts powdered ginger, pepper (ground black), long-pepper, celery and cumin (seeds), and salt (rock). Swallow 1 tsp. of this mixture when you eat your 1st bite at every meal.

Avoid: Stress, cold meals, scattered eating times, snacking.

A must do when practicing Ayurveda involves seeing an Ayurvedic practitioner. I must advise you to visit one. They can help you and diagnose your issues. I am just here to give you the basic knowledge and stepping stones you need in order to take the imbalance in your life and rebalance it.

There are an immense number of treatments, therapies, and techniques available and it is difficult for the inexperienced to pick the proper one. Then, some of the time, you will need to have someone else preform the therapy anyway. Pick your Ayurvedic practitioner just as carefully as you would a doctor, there are many to choose from wherever you live.

Ayurvedic practitioners will probably recommend more than one treatment. Most of the time they will prescribe everyday activities and treatments for home for your daily schedule/dincharya, along with more infrequent or seasonal/ritucharya treatments. These include, but are not limited to:

- Shirodhara

  This therapy uses dripped oil on the head, between the eyes (forehead), where the third eye would be. The particular oil, the amount of times this treatment is performed, and how long the treatment lasts depends on the reason for the treatment. That is why it is important to find a great practitioner.

- Dietary modifications

  Diet plays a huge part in the Ayurvedic perspective. Foods are the fuel for your body and mind and can easily disrupt balance. They are part of treating a problem, recovering from an issue, and continually working on a disease if necessary. Your dietary/nutritional plan can be developed to meet you exact individual needs by an experienced practitioner. They use 6 tastes to form their plans:

  - Sweets: are nourishing for tissue and encourages strength

  - Sour foods: fuel power in the digestive system

- Salty foods: keep electrolyte balance in water

- Strong foods: aid in digesting and absorbing foods

- Bitter foods: help to encourage the other 5 tastes

- Astringent foods: aid in absorbing of nutrients

- Massage: There are Ayurvedic massage therapists who are supervised and under-go training provided by practitioners. They will use specific oils depending on the practitioner's recommendations.

- Panchakarma: this is a complex detox program. It rids the body of ama (toxins). It may consist of massage-therapy, steaming, forced throwing up (vamana), forced elimination (virechana) using laxatives, blood-letting, and nose treatments (nasya). Also included is usually a diet plan with herbal supplementation and a revision of everyday activities. It is extreme and should always be undergone under the care of a well-trained practitioner.

- Herbal treatments: they are concocted based upon tastes (ras), how potent they are (virya), and what effect they have once they have been digested (vipak). It is part of the science of Ayurveda health care and extensive knowledge of the herbs and how they alter the body and the emotions/ and thinking. Herbal treatments should only be concocted by a great practitioner.

What goes into a practitioner's diagnosis and treatment plan?

We, as westerners, go to a doctor when we feel sick. They then try to figure out what we have and treat the cause or sometimes just the symptoms. Usually the same prescription drugs, amount of toxic-medicine, and possibly procedure is given in the same way to many people just because they have the same illness or symptoms.

Under the Ayurvedic healthcare system, the diagnosis and prescription/treatments are not only based on the actual illness and severity; they also consider the patient as an individual as well. They treat the illness by custom tailoring it to every different patient.

Ayurvedic medicine teaches that every single person has the tools and energies inside of them that, with the proper guidance, will enable them to achieve health through balance. That is why Ayurevedic practitioners strive to use treatments that will boost deficiencies and decrease excess in the body. The remedies and therapies are simply used to enable the body to better heal itself, as opposed to western medicines taking up the healing.

The practitioner comes to these conclusions after a thorough exam. What happens during an exam? I am so glad you asked!

They will ask you a lot of questions. Be prepared to answer in detail. Not only will they ask about your past health, but most will ask about many different areas of your life: diet, your family and relationships, your emotional and mental health, your occupation, and so on.

The exams are broken up into 3 different areas:

- Darshan/Observing: They will check the body, noticing the way the patient moves, their body-shape/type, tone of skin, eye color, nose, and the condition of the mouth, hair and also toe/finger nails.
- Touching/Sparsha: They will press and tap on different areas and listen to the inner workings of the organs. They will pay attention to the heartbeat/rate, tongue, pattern of speech, and fingernails.

- Asking/ Prashna: They will ask about your issues and what you are experiencing as far as symptoms. Practitioners also need to know how long your illness has been going on and how bad the illness has become. They will want details of current and prior emotional and mental health issues.

Ayurveda is such a wonderful practice. It takes into consideration each individual and what they need in order to achieve optimum health. It is a healthcare system that is concerned with and based around holistic health and wellness.

Chapter 5 Ayurvedic Recipes for Wellness and Balance

When I first heard of Ayurveda, I thought, as most people do that Ayurveda is strictly vegetarian. Well, most of the recipes do not include meat, but that is for general overall health and not just on principle. There are Ayurvedic recipes that include meat, but these are intended for specific uses in order to rebalance something in the body that is out of balance.

Ayurveda does not ban alcoholic beverages or meats. They are intended for specific medicinal purposes. They also have the tendency, when ingested in large amounts or on a consistent basis, to throw off the balance of the body. They are harsher and more difficult for the body to process.

Generally speaking, Ayurveda pushes a mostly vegetarian diet and recommends staying away from alcohol, for the purpose of keeping a good mind and body balance. There is no rule saying that you cannot eat these occasionally, just remember what your body and mind need in order to operate at their best.

Vatta Breakfast

Pancakes

- ½ teaspoon baking powder
- 1 Tablespoon salted butter
- ¼ teaspoon each: cardamom, ginger and nutmeg
- ½ cup shelled pistachios
- 1 Tablespoon sugar (raw)
- 1/8 tsp salt (mineral)
- 1 cup flour (spelt)
- ½ teaspoon vanilla extract
- 1 cup water

1. Chop pistachios in food processor
2. All dry ingredients, mix with fork in a bowl
3. Mix all wet ingredients in another bowl
4. Combine all ingredients
5. Cook on a griddle or skillet over medium heat (preheat the skillet) until the pancake tans on bottom and bubbles on top
6. Flip and cook other side for 2-3 min

Green Frittata

- ¼ teaspoon pepper
- 6 eggs
- 1 teaspoon of both: fresh parsley and thyme
- ½ teaspoon oregano
- ¼ teaspoon salt

1. Set oven to 350
2. Chop up herbs and mix with all other ingredient in a mixing bowl.
3. Whisk eggs
4. Grease a cast-iron skillet and heat to medium.
5. Add mixture when hot (should sizzle)
6. Take off of the heat and put the skillet straight into the oven for 20 min.

Pitta Breakfast

Smoothie

- 2 cups of bananas
- ¼ teaspoon cardamom
- ½ lime
- 1 cup of coconut water or spring water

  -Mix all in blender till smooth

Almonds meal

- 2 Tablespoons Almonds raw
- ¼ teaspoon each: cardamom and cinnamon
- 1 teaspoon each: maple syrup and ghee
- 1 cup milk (or almond milk)
- 1/3 cup oats

1. Soak almonds all night
2. Peel off skin in the morning

3. Put almonds and oats in coffee grinder and grind
4. Put the oats, almonds and all other ingredients in a saucepan
5. If you are experiencing dryness, double the milk
6. Heat to medium-high until it , stir it the whole time
7. Turn to low and simmer

Kapha Breakfast

Grapefruit with fennel

- 1.5 teaspoons fennel seeds
- 1 peeled grapefruit separated

1. Put fennel seeds in coffee grinder or food processer until it becomes a powder
2. Sprinkle over grapefruit

Breakfast Tea

- ¼ in. piece of ginger
- 1 teaspoon honey
- ¼ lemon

-Mash the ginger with a mortar/pestle. Put boiling water in mortar, stir, then put in cup. Mix in other ingredients.

Lunch Vata

Squash Soup

¼ teaspoon pepper

- 4 cups butternut squash
- 1 teaspoons fennel seeds
- 2 garlic cloves
- ½ in. piece of ginger
- ½ lime
- 2 Tablespoons EVOO
- ¼ teaspoon salt
- 4 cups water
- ½ cup onion
- Peel entire squash

1. Chop up onion and brown in evoo over medium, when almost done add ginger/garlic. Cook for thirty seconds
2. Add all other ingredients.
3. Bring it to a boil and then turn to medium for twenty min. stirring occasionally. Make sure squash is tender

Zucchini Rice

- 1/3 cup rice-basmati
- ¼ teaspoon pepper
- 2 carrots
- ¼ inch ginger
- 4 cups water
- 1 TBSP sunflower oil
- 1 cup chopped zucchini
- ¼ teaspoon salt

1. Boil water
2. Chop up zucchini and carrots. Grate the ginger up well.
3. Put everything in water and bring back to a boil
4. Turn down, simmer and cover until rice is ready

<u>Lunch Pitta</u>

Mung-kitchari

- 1 cup rice (basmati)

- 1/3 cup chopped cilantro
- 1/3 cup flaked coconut
- 2 Tablespoons Ghee
- 1 inch ginger
- ½ cup mung-bean
- ¼ teaspoon salt
- ½ teaspoon turmeric
- 6 cups of water

1. Wash mung and rice in separate strainers
2. Soak mung for an hour or two and drain well
3. Add ½ cup water, ginger/cilantro/coconut in a food processor until it turns to liquid
4. Heat a sauce pan to medium with ghee, add food processor mix with turmeric/salt
5. Stir all and heat to boil, stirring the whole time
6. Mix in rice
7. Add mung and water, return to boil uncovered 5 min
8. Cover with lid tilted, turn down to simmer for 30 min

Lunch Pitta

Warm Carrot Soup

- 4 carrots
- ½ teaspoon fennel seed
- 1 inch of fresh ginger
- 1 pound of kale
- ½ of a lime
- 1 Tablespoon sunflower oil

1. Wash and chop kale and the carrots. Put in a large saucepan, cover with water.
2. Bring to a boil until kale is soft.

Date Roasted Rice

- 1 cup rice (basmati)
- 1/8 teaspoon pepper
- ¼ teaspoon cardamom
- ¼ teaspoon cinnamon
- 4 dried dates

- 1 Tablespoon ghee
- 1/8 teaspoon salt
- 3 cups of water

1. Chop the dates up really well
2. Boil water and add all into a pot
3. Cook for 20 min covered

Lunch Kapha

Savory White Beans

- 1/8 teaspoon pepper
- ¼ teaspoons of cumin
- ½ of a lemon
- 2 Tablespoons EVOO
- 1/3 cup fresh parsley
- ¼ teaspoon salt
- 1 cup white beans

1. Let the beans soak all night.
2. Rinse and drain the beans

3. Put all beans in a large sauce pan to boil until they are tender

4. Drain the water, put in the lemon juice/salt/pepper and mix

5. Wait 10 minutes and mix all ingredients

6. Chill

Herbed Tomato Salad

- 1 cup chopped kale
- 1 Tablespoon ACV
- ¼ cup of basil
- 3 TBSP EVOO
- ¼ teaspoon oregano
- 1 teaspoon raw sugar
- ½ cup onion (red is best)
- 1/8 teaspoon fresh thyme
- 4 tomatoes

1. Chop up tomato, mix with other items and pour over tomatoes

Lunch Pitta

Asparagus Rice

- 1 cup of asparagus
- 1 cup rice (basmati)
- ¼ teaspoon salt
- 1 Tablespoon sunflower oil
- 3 cups of water

1. Sautee mushroom in oil on a frying pan (space 1 in. apart)
2. Chop asparagus into 1 in. pieces
3. Put the rest of the oil in a large saucepan and sautee asparagus (it will turn bright when done)
4. Mix in rice and mushrooms until oil coats rice
5. Add all ingredients, turn to high and bring to boil
6. Turn down to low, cover and simmer for 20 min

Dinner Vata

Nutty Citrus Rice

- 1 cup rice (basmati)
- ¾ cup cashew
- ½ teaspoon cumin
- ¼ cup ghee
- 2 Lemons
- ½ teaspoon mustard seeds
- Pinch salt
- 1 cup of peas
- ½ teaspoon turmeric

1. Roast the cumin and mustard on frying pan until popping occurs
2. In alternate pot roast rice and nuts in ghee until they are light brown
3. Mix in 2 cups of water, boil, cover, turn down to low and simmer for twenty five min
4. Add peas, cooking for ten more min
5. Squeeze the lemon over the rice

6. Put in a bowl

Spiced Yams and Mushrooms

- ¼ teaspoon each: pepper, cinnamon
- 3 garlic cloves
- 1 cup of mushrooms
- 2 Tablespoons EVOO
- 1 teaspoon rosemary
- Pinch salt
- 4 cups Yams
- ¼ onion

1. Boil yams with spices/water, put on lid and simmer
2. Sautee mushrooms, separated by an inch
3. Add onion and keep cooking until they are clear
4. Put in garlic for less than one min and then dump all in with yams
5. Simmer until yams are tender

Dinner Pitta

Sweet Coconut Potato Soup

- 1 cup coconut milk
- ½ inch of ginger
- ¼ of a lime
- Pinch salt
- 2 Tablespoons stinging nettles
- 2 cups of sweet potato
- 3 cups of water

1. Squeeze the lime into a sauce pan, grate ginger in and add all ingredients into the pot (just not nettles)
2. Boil then turn to a simmer
3. When potatoes are tender, put in a bender
4. Add nettles

-

Potatoes n' Peas

- 3 Potatoes, cut into chunks (russet)
- 1 c. of peas
- 1 Onion (chop)
- 1 large tomato (chop)
- 1 bay leaf
- 1 teaspoon each turmeric and cumin
- ¼ teaspoon salt
- ¼ cup of water
- 2 Tablespoons EVOO
- Prepared basmati rice according to package

1. Using a non-stick pan heat oil to medium-high, throw in cumin and bay
2. When it is done splattering, mix in onion
3. Brown until onions become clear then add tomato
4. Soften tomato and then put in all of the spices for 1 min
5. Mix in potatoes, reducing the heat to low
6. Mix in your water. Put a lid of and simmer 15 min or until potatoes are soft

7. Mix in peas and re-cover for 10 more minutes
8. Serve with prepared plain basmati rice

****

Dinner Kapha

Corn Chowder

- ¼ teaspoon pepper
- ½ cup chopped celery
- 1/8 teaspoon chipotle-chili
- 2 cups of corn
- ½ teaspoon curry (powdered)
- ½ of a lime
- 2 potatoes
- Pinch salt
- 2 Tablespoons sunflower oil
- 1 large tomato

1. Chop up tomatoes and potatoes. Mix with celery, corn and in a large pot

2. Cover with water and boil
3. While waiting you can sautee spices in oil, then toss in the onions and brown them
4. Add to the soup

****

Corn Mung-fritters

- Pinch pepper
- ½ cup corn flour
- 1/8 teaspoon fenugreek
- 2 teaspoons ghee
- ¼ lemon
- ½ cup mung beans
- 1 cup of fresh parsley
- 2 Tablespoons chopped onion
- Pinch salt

1. Put mung in coffee grinder and grind.
2. Mix with corn, salt and seasoning.

3. Add onion/parsley/ lemon with 1 cup of water, soaking 30 min
4. Fry all in ghee

Conclusion

Thank you again for purchasing this booklet!

I hope this book was able to help you to give you, as a Westerner and a beginner, a general understanding of Ayurveda and its usefulness as a practical healthcare system to achieve true health and wellness by balancing your mind and body with the world around you.

It is simple to start. You have the tools. Why waste another day with your body and mind in a state of imbalance, toxicity, and possibly chaos? You have everything it takes within yourself to achieve holistic health, and Ayurveda has the tools to give your body the boost it needs in order to make this happen.

I encourage you to take the next step and visit an Ayurvedic practitioner. They can help you delve into this lifestyle. I hope I have sparked your interest just as my yoga instructor did for me years ago. If only I had heard earlier! Do not waste another day in a state of health that you do not need to be in. Rebalance yourself now and live the life you have always desired.

Thank you and good luck!

Ayurvedic Resources I recommend:

If you want to keep investigating Ayurveda in India, do it! I am sure you will love it! However, you can stay where you are and learn more about Ayurveda using my favorite resources. The good thing about our Western culture is that we invented the internet and social media. Let's use it to our advantage and to our wellness and health.

Doctor Vasant Lad (I really recommend his seminars!)

http://www.youtube.com/user/AyurvedicInstitute

Psychetruth (Nutrition, Massage, Wellness, Balance)

http://www.youtube.com/user/psychetruth

Ayurveda, The Art of Being (A wonderful documentary that is available on youtube)

****

Bonus Chapter

The preview of my book: *Feng Shui for Wellness and Wealth*

The name Feng Shui is a combination of two words: *Feng* (wind) and *Shui* (water). These two elements are seen as being vital to human survival and thus, are carriers of 'chi' or life force. Thus, the practice of Feng Shui involves designing environments in order to improve the flow of chi.

One of the basic things that you can do to start the process of Feng Shui in your home or office is to remove the clutter from these spaces. When your home or office is filled with possessions that you do not use, need or want, it blocks the natural flow of chi through these spaces. Of course, decluttering these spaces is difficult, particularly if the clutter has been allowed to build up over a long time. But it can be done.

One way to approach 'decluttering', so that it won't be overwhelming, is to do it step by step. You can devote thirty minutes a session to removing the clutter and then stop when the time is up. Continue next time with another session until the room has been cleared, and then move on to the next one. You can also make the task more pleasant by bringing in a sense of positive energy to the task. Open the windows to allow fresh air to come in, and then play some soothing music while you are working. Work with aromatherapy oils or natural incenses to bring some pleasant and harmonious fragrances. Before you know it, you'll be done with the task without feeling heavy or unpleasant, Once you have removed all the clutter from your environment, you'll be surprised at how much lighter you feel and how you seem to have more energy when you're in that space.

Imagine that your flat/ house/ office is a living organism. Imagine that it is not feeling well at all, you can even imagine that it is disease-stricken. Keep repeating to yourself:

I am a healer. I restore balance where there is imbalance!

As soon as you remove all the clutter (it stands for bacteria in our visualization technique) our space will be healed and attracting only good energies that we need so much.

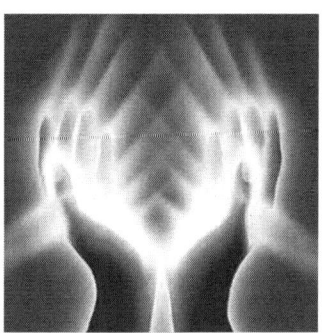

Yes! You will be attracting your personal and professional success with your own hands!

Using Feng Shui principles in your office is very important in order to ensure that your personal *chi* is in harmony with your surroundings, which will help you become more efficient and more productive. Unless you have your own office, there are only a limited number of things that you can do to arrange the furnishings in your work space, Nevertheless, there are some things that you can do to create better Feng Shui.

For your cubicle:

- First of all, organize your work space to ensure that it is neat. For example, don't leave files that you are not using lying around, but instead return them to the proper cabinet. Avoid having excess clutter on your desk. In particular, remove old items that are no longer useful or things that carry bad memories, such as reports that were rejected.

- As much as possible, move your desk in such a way that you can see the entrance to your cubicle. Place a poster of an earth element such as a forest or canyon on the wall behind you. If you cannot move your desk, place a small mirror on it in such a way that you can see if someone is approaching.

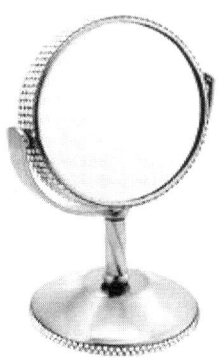

Mirrors play an important part in an intelligent Feng Shui-friendly design.

- Place a plant in a red pot, such as a money tree or a small bamboo, at the east side of your desk to energize your work space. Avoid sharp plants such as cacti since they generate bad chi. In addition, you can place good fortune symbols such as a dragon, turtle or unicorn, around your cubicle or desk.

- Put your computer on the west side of your desk to encourage creativity or on the southeast side to promote increased income.

- Place red objects on your desk at the south corner to ensure that you are recognized for your good work. Alternately, you can place a crystal in the south to achieve the same effect.

For your office:

- Make sure that when a visitor enters your office, they see something pleasant such as a healthy plant, since this creates positive chi. You can also put a small fountain near the entrance since this can help improve your mood as well as helping generate more income.

- Don't allow clutter or defective equipment to stay in your office. Have them removed. If they cannot be removed at once, place them somewhere, such as a closet, where they are not visible. For the same reason, you should have electrical cords and cables neatly tucked away since they create a sense of disorder.

- Place equipment such as computers and telephones in the southeast (or wealth) area to encourage increased business to come in.

- If possible, place an aquarium in the north corner of your office to promote increased business success. Put black and blue fish in it since they absorb negative *chi*.

- Don't place mirrors in the reception area since these will reflect *chi* back out of your office.

Feng Shui And The Law Of Attraction:

One of the most important tools in Feng Shui is the compass since you can use it to determine the different directions in your office. Every direction has a different type of energy associated with it and by placing the proper objects in these positions; you can promote the desired effect.

North: career

South: Reputation

West: Creativity and children

East: Family and health

Northeast: Knowledge

Northwest: Helpful people and travel

Southeast: Wealth

Southwest: Love and relationships

I suggest you take a piece of paper and write down all the areas of your life that needs improvement, e.g:

>-I want to travel to exotic countries at least twice a year;

>-I want to live a healthy and balanced life;

>-I want to attract more romance in my life and attract the opposite sex like a magnet.

Now analyze the current organization of your house or apartment. Before we actually get started on specific Feng Shui steps for different areas of your life and your house, I would like you to use your intuition. Let's say that you are looking for wealth and abundance: how does the Southeast part of your apartment or office reflect what you want? Maybe it's full of clutter and just totally disorganized? I strongly suggest you do this exercise just using your intuition and common sense. Write down your thoughts and then compare them with my instructions from the next chapters of this book. Also, ask yourself how you could improve the given part of your house or office simply following your intuition. A really fun task to do, so make sure you don't skip it!

From my own experience:

When I originally got started on Feng Shui, I wanted to attract more romance into my life. I therefore revised the Southwest part of my apartment, especially my bedroom. I had been making a horrible mistake of accumulating all the 'old bachelor's stuff' as well as 'little boy's stuff', like for example: some awards from Junior High and pictures from my favorite football matches that I watched with my buddies. No wonder that all the females were avoiding me. I was making it obvious to the Universe: I want to carry on the way I live and just hang out with my male friends and watch football!

It wasn't until I removed all the clutter that had been accumulating there for years and made the whole area clean. I simply used my imagination as this is what my Feng Shui coach suggested. He asked me: *If you had a girlfriend or a lover how would you re-organize your flat/ bedroom to create an atmosphere for lovers rather than for school boys or old bachelors?*

What I did was simple: I set up a mini table with a CD player and I purchased lots of relaxation and massage music CDs. I also got cinnamon incense sticks and got the hottest aromatherapy oils for lovers that possibly exist: ylang ylang and cedar wood. I just knew that this new 'deco' would show the Universe what I wanted. I also felt that I was getting enough confidence- I began to believe that I was a new Casanova. I even got a few books on Tantric Sex and Natural Aphrodisiacs and exposed them in my 'Love and Romance' corner. Then I would gradually transform myself from a lonely and depressed man to a man that could actually get to enjoy female company and touch whenever he wanted...

If you enjoyed reading this free preview, you will love my book:

Feng Shui For Wellness And Wealth: Simple Feng Shui Tricks For Personal And Professional Success- Health, Money and Happiness With Feng Shui Tips.

Simply search for it on Amazon. I hope you will enjoy it!

James Adler's Books:

Success Secrets: Change Your Life With Neuro-Linguistic Programming. NLP Techniques for Personal and Professional Success and Lifestyle Transformation

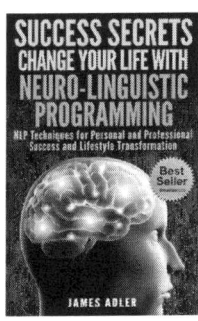

NLP For Fast Weight Loss

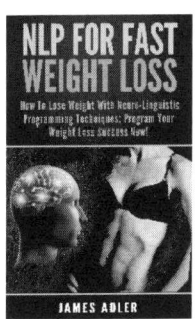

Alkaline Weight Loss and Wellness

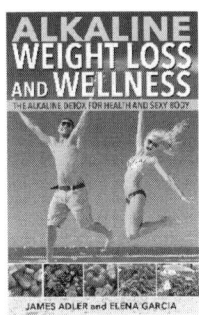

Paleo Lifestyle for Healthy Weight. The Paleo Diet for Weight Loss, Health and Vitality. Transform Yourself With Delicious Paleo Recipes!

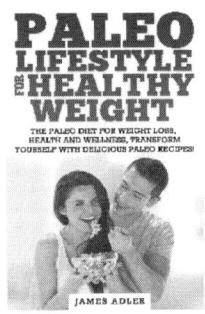

Great reads from my fellow authors:

Visit our facebook page:

www.facebook.com/holisticwellnessbooks

...and be the first one to find out about free and bargain books and eBooks related to health and wellness.

Thank You again for your time and interest in our work.

James Adler and Holistic Wellness Books

Printed in Great Britain
by Amazon.co.uk, Ltd.,
Marston Gate.